Asthma Alchemy

Transforming Your Lung Health.

Copyright Notice

Disclaimer

This book falls within the realm of nonfiction in the field of health. The information presented here is intended solely for general informational purposes and should not be considered a replacement for professional medical advice, diagnosis, or treatment. It is imperative to always seek guidance from a qualified healthcare provider or physician regarding any inquiries you may have about a medical condition. Please do not disregard professional medical advice or delay seeking it based on the content found in this book.

Contents

Introduction

Welcome to "Asthma Alchemy: Transforming Your Lung Health." Within the pages of this book lies a journey of empowerment, understanding, and transformation—an exploration of the intricate art and science of managing asthma.

Asthma is a condition that touches millions of lives around the world, from children to seniors, athletes to artists. It is a condition that, at times, can feel like a relentless adversary, diminishing our capacity to breathe freely and live fully. Yet, within the challenges it presents, there exists a remarkable opportunity—an alchemy of sorts.

This book is your guide through this alchemical process—a journey that takes you from the initial spark of knowledge to the forging of a path to better lung health. In these chapters, we will delve into the inner workings of asthma, understanding its triggers, the role of medications, and the power of lifestyle modifications. We will explore the transformative potential of breathing techniques, the holistic approaches of natural remedies, and the importance of creating an asthma-friendly environment.

As you embark on this journey, remember that asthma alchemy is not a one-size-fits-all process. Each person's experience with asthma is unique, and so too will be your approach to its management. Whether you are navigating the challenges of childhood asthma, embracing adulthood with asthma, or facing the nuances of senior asthma, there is something within these pages for everyone.

Our aim is to empower you, the reader, to transform your relationship with asthma. By arming you with knowledge, and offering practical strategies, we hope to shift the perception of asthma from a burden to an opportunity—a catalyst for better lung health and a fuller, more fulfilling life.

So, let us begin this transformative journey together, as we unlock the secrets of "Asthma Alchemy" and embark on a path to breathing easier, living healthier, and discovering the alchemical art of transforming your lung health.

Chapter 1

Understanding Asthma: Unraveling the Mysteries

Asthma is a chronic inflammatory condition of the airways, characterized by recurrent episodes of wheezing, breathlessness, chest tightness, and coughing. These symptoms can range from mild to severe, and they often occur in episodes or attacks. Asthma attacks can be triggered by various factors, making it a condition that demands constant vigilance and proactive management.

The Inflammatory Process

At the heart of asthma lies inflammation. In individuals with asthma, the airways become overly sensitive to certain triggers, such as allergens, respiratory infections, irritants, and exercise. When exposed to these triggers, the airways can become inflamed and constrict, causing the classic symptoms of asthma.

Understanding the Triggers

Asthma triggers are varied and can differ from person to person. Common triggers include:

1. **Allergens:** Allergens are substances that can trigger allergic reactions in individuals who are sensitive or allergic to them. Allergens are a well-known and common trigger for asthma symptoms, and understanding their role is crucial in managing and preventing asthma attacks. Allergens can be categorized into several types, including pollen, dust mites, pet dander, mold spores, and certain foods. When individuals with asthma come into contact with these allergens, their immune system can overreact, leading to an allergic response.

Asthma symptoms can be triggered when allergens are inhaled. For example, pollen from trees, grasses, or weeds can be inhaled and irritate the airways, especially in people with allergic asthma. Sensitization occurs when the immune system becomes hypersensitive to specific allergens, leading to an exaggerated response upon subsequent exposure.

When allergens enter the respiratory system, the immune system releases chemicals such as histamines and leukotrienes. These chemicals can cause inflammation and swelling of the airway walls, leading to bronchoconstriction, which narrows the airways and makes it difficult to breathe.

Allergens can directly trigger asthma symptoms. For example, dust mites in bedding or pet dander in the home can provoke an asthma attack. Individuals with asthma may notice a worsening of symptoms when exposed to specific allergens, and these symptoms can vary in severity.

Some allergens, like pollen, have a seasonal pattern. This means that asthma symptoms in individuals with allergic asthma can worsen during certain times of the year when specific allergens are prevalent. This is known as seasonal asthma.

2. **Respiratory Infections:** Respiratory infections, such as viral infections, bacterial infections, and even fungal infections, can serve as significant triggers for asthma exacerbations. These infections can worsen asthma symptoms and lead to acute asthma attacks. Here's how respiratory infections can act as triggers for asthma:

Respiratory infections typically cause inflammation in the airways. In asthma, the airways are already inflamed, and this inflammation is further exacerbated during an infection. This increased inflammation can lead to a worsening of asthma symptoms, including increased bronchoconstriction and mucus production.

Infections can cause the muscles surrounding the airways to contract, leading to bronchoconstriction or narrowing of the airways. This narrowing makes it harder for individuals with asthma to breathe and can result in coughing, wheezing, and shortness of breath.

In response to infection, the airway lining may produce excess mucus. This can further obstruct the airways, making it difficult for air to flow freely and exacerbating asthma symptoms.

Viral respiratory infections, especially rhinovirus (the most common cause of the common cold), are well-known triggers for asthma exacerbations. Other viruses, such as influenza and respiratory syncytial virus (RSV), can also worsen asthma symptoms. In some cases, viral infections may directly infect the lower respiratory tract, which can be especially problematic for individuals with asthma.

While less common than viral infections, bacterial respiratory infections, such as bronchitis or pneumonia, can also trigger asthma symptoms. These infections can lead to increased airway inflammation and mucus production.

Fungal infections, particularly in individuals with compromised immune systems, can affect the respiratory system and worsen asthma symptoms. Allergic bronchopulmonary aspergillosis (ABPA) is an example of a fungal infection that can exacerbate asthma.

Respiratory infections can make individuals with asthma more sensitive to other triggers, such as allergens or irritants. This heightened sensitivity can persist even after the infection has resolved, making asthma management more challenging.

3.   **Irritants:** Irritants are substances or environmental factors that can trigger or exacerbate asthma symptoms in individuals with asthma. Unlike allergens, which provoke an allergic response, irritants can directly irritate the airways, leading to inflammation and bronchoconstriction.

Common irritants that can trigger asthma symptoms include:

- **Tobacco Smoke:** Exposure to secondhand smoke or active smoking is a well-known asthma trigger. The chemicals in tobacco smoke can irritate the airways and worsen inflammation.

- **Air Pollution:** Outdoor air pollution, including particulate matter (PM2.5 and PM10) and ground-level ozone, can irritate the airways and lead to asthma exacerbations. Indoor air pollution from sources like wood-burning stoves or cooking fumes can also be problematic.

- **Strong Odors:** Strong odors, such as perfumes, cleaning products, paint fumes, and scented candles, can trigger asthma symptoms in some individuals.

- **Volatile Organic Compounds (VOCs):** VOCs emitted by various household products and building materials, including formaldehyde, can irritate the airways.

- **Cold Air:** Breathing in cold, dry air can cause airway constriction in some people with asthma.

- **Chemical Irritants:** Exposure to workplace chemicals, industrial fumes, or cleaning agents can irritate the airways and trigger asthma symptoms.

When irritants come into contact with the airways, they can lead to an inflammatory response. This inflammation can result in airway swelling, increased mucus production, and bronchoconstriction, making it difficult to breathe.

Irritants can trigger both immediate and delayed asthma responses. Some individuals may experience rapid onset of symptoms upon exposure to irritants, while others may have a delayed reaction. Prolonged or repeated exposure to irritants can have a cumulative effect on asthma symptoms. Over time, ongoing exposure to irritants can lead to chronic airway inflammation and more frequent asthma exacerbations.

4. **Exercise:** Exercise-induced bronchoconstriction (EIB), also known as exercise-induced asthma (EIA), is a condition in which physical activity triggers asthma symptoms or worsens existing asthma. However, it's essential to note that exercise should not discourage individuals with asthma from staying active. With proper management and precautions, people with asthma can engage in physical activities and enjoy the many benefits of exercise.

During exercise, individuals typically breathe more rapidly and deeply, which can lead to the cooling and drying of the airways. In people with EIB, this process can trigger the release of inflammatory substances, such as histamines and leukotrienes, causing bronchoconstriction and inflammation in the airways.

The symptoms of EIB can include coughing, wheezing, shortness of breath, chest tightness, and decreased exercise tolerance. These symptoms usually begin during or shortly after exercise and may persist for a variable period.

EIB is distinct from asthma triggered by allergens or irritants. It primarily occurs during or after physical exertion and is often not related to exposure to allergens or irritants.

EIB can affect individuals with asthma, as well as those without a history of asthma. It's estimated that a significant portion of individuals with asthma experiences EIB, and even some elite athletes may develop exercise-induced symptoms.

5. **Emotional Factors:** Stress and strong emotions can lead to shallow breathing and potentially trigger asthma symptoms.

The Role of Genetics

The role of genetics in asthma is a subject of significant scientific interest and research. While asthma is a complex condition influenced by both genetic and environmental factors, understanding the genetic component is crucial for gaining insights into its underlying mechanisms, heritability, and potential avenues for personalized treatment and prevention. Here's an overview of the role of genetics in asthma:

1. **Heritability:** Asthma tends to run in families, and individuals with a family history of asthma or other allergic conditions (like hay fever or eczema) are at a higher risk of developing asthma themselves. This familial clustering suggests a genetic predisposition to the condition. Studies of twins have estimated that the heritability of asthma is approximately 35-95%, indicating a significant genetic component.

2. **Candidate Genes:** Researchers have identified several candidate genes associated with asthma susceptibility. These genes are involved in various aspects of immune response, airway inflammation, and airway hyper responsiveness. Some notable genes include those related to:

- **Immune System:** Variations in genes that regulate immune responses, such as interleukins (e.g., IL-4, IL-13) and tumor necrosis factor alpha (TNF-α), have been linked to asthma susceptibility.

- **Airway Inflammation:** Genes involved in the inflammatory response, such as those encoding for leukotrienes and prostaglandins, have been implicated in asthma.

- **Bronchial Smooth Muscle Function:** Certain genes associated with bronchial smooth muscle contraction and relaxation, such as those encoding for beta-2 adrenergic receptors, are relevant in asthma.

3. **Genome-Wide Association Studies (GWAS):** Advances in genetic research have led to large-scale genome-wide association studies (GWAS) that aim to identify specific genetic variants associated with asthma. These studies have revealed numerous single nucleotide polymorphisms (SNPs) and genetic markers linked to asthma susceptibility. GWAS have also highlighted the importance of gene-environment interactions, showing that certain genetic variants may increase the risk of asthma when combined with specific environmental exposures, such as tobacco smoke or allergens.

4.   Heterogeneity: Asthma is a heterogeneous condition, meaning it can present differently in different individuals. Genetics plays a role in this heterogeneity by influencing the type and severity of asthma symptoms, as well as the response to treatments. Some genetic variants are associated with more severe forms of asthma, while others may be related to milder, intermittent asthma.

5. Personalized Medicine: Understanding the genetic basis of asthma holds promise for the development of personalized treatments. Genetic information can help healthcare providers tailor asthma management strategies, including the choice of medications and dosages. For example, certain genetic variants may predict a better response to specific asthma medications like bronchodilators or corticosteroids.

Symptoms and Diagnosis

Asthma is a chronic respiratory condition that can vary in severity and presentation among individuals. Common symptoms of asthma include:

1. **Wheezing:** Wheezing is a high-pitched whistling sound that occurs during breathing, especially when exhaling. It results from the narrowing of the airways and is a hallmark symptom of asthma.

2. **Coughing:** Persistent or recurrent coughing, particularly at night or in the early morning, is a common symptom. Coughing may be dry or produce mucus.

3. **Shortness of Breath:** Individuals with asthma often experience difficulty breathing, which can manifest as a feeling of breathlessness or tightness in the chest.

4. **Chest Tightness:** Many people with asthma describe a sensation of tightness or discomfort in the chest. This tightness is often associated with exacerbations of asthma symptoms.

5. **Increased Mucus Production:** The inflammation in the airways can lead to increased mucus production, which may contribute to coughing and breathing difficulties.

6. **Symptoms That Vary:** Asthma symptoms can vary over time, with periods of exacerbation (asthma attacks) and periods of relative symptom relief (remission). Triggers like allergens, respiratory infections, or exposure to irritants can worsen symptoms.

7. **Exercise-Induced Symptoms:** Some individuals with asthma experience exercise-induced bronchoconstriction, where physical activity triggers or exacerbates asthma symptoms.

8. **Nighttime Symptoms:** Asthma symptoms often worsen at night, which can disrupt sleep and lead to fatigue during the day.

Diagnosis of Asthma:

Diagnosing asthma involves a comprehensive evaluation by a healthcare provider. The diagnostic process typically includes the following steps:

1. **Medical History:** The healthcare provider will gather a detailed medical history, including information about symptoms, their frequency, and any potential triggers or patterns. Family history of asthma or allergic conditions may also be discussed.

2. **Physical Examination:** A physical examination can help assess lung function and rule out other respiratory conditions. During the examination, the healthcare provider will listen to the patient's breathing using a stethoscope.

3. **Lung Function Tests:** Lung function tests, such as spirometry and peak flow measurements, are essential for diagnosing and assessing the severity of asthma. Spirometry measures how much air a person can exhale forcefully and how quickly they can do so. Peak flow measurements track changes in airflow over time.

4. **Allergy Testing:** Allergy tests may be performed to identify specific allergens that could be triggering asthma symptoms. Skin prick tests and blood tests are common methods used for allergy testing.

5. **Bronchial Challenge Test:** In some cases, a bronchial challenge test may be conducted to assess airway responsiveness. This test involves inhaling a substance that can trigger airway constriction, and then measuring the lung function response.

6. **Chest X-ray or CT Scan:** These imaging studies are not typically used for asthma diagnosis but may be performed if there is uncertainty about the diagnosis or to rule out other lung conditions.

7. **Asthma Diary:** Keeping a daily record of symptoms and peak flow measurements can help healthcare providers evaluate asthma control over time.

8. **Asthma Action Plan:** Once diagnosed, individuals with asthma should work with their healthcare provider to develop a personalized asthma action

plan. This plan outlines steps to take for symptom management, exacerbation prevention, and emergency situations.

Asthma diagnosis requires a careful evaluation of the patient's clinical history, physical examination findings, and lung function tests. It is essential for accurately identifying asthma, determining its severity, and tailoring an appropriate treatment plan to manage the condition effectively.

The Future of Asthma

Ongoing research seeks to unravel the complexities of asthma, with the goal of improving diagnosis, treatment, and ultimately finding a cure. Personalized medicine and targeted therapies hold promise for more effective asthma management. Additionally, efforts to reduce asthma disparities and improve access to care are essential for better outcomes among underserved populations.

The nature of asthma is complex and multifaceted, encompassing genetic predispositions, environmental triggers, inflammatory processes, and a wide range of symptoms. Understanding this complex condition is essential for individuals living with asthma, their caregivers, and healthcare providers. With proper management and ongoing research, we can continue to improve the lives of those affected by asthma, transforming it from a challenging condition into one that is manageable and well-controlled.

The Causes of Asthma

Asthma is a complex and multifactorial respiratory condition, and its exact causes are not fully understood. Instead, asthma is believed to result from a combination of genetic, environmental, and immunological factors. Here's a breakdown of the various factors that contribute to the development of asthma:

1. Genetic Factors:

- **Family History:** Individuals with a family history of asthma or allergic conditions like hay fever (allergic rhinitis) or eczema (atopic dermatitis) are at a higher risk of developing asthma. This suggests a genetic predisposition to the condition.

- **Genetic Variants:** Certain genetic variations or polymorphisms have been associated with an increased susceptibility to asthma. These variations may affect the immune system's response to allergens and irritants.

2. Environmental Factors:

- **Allergens:** Exposure to allergens such as pollen, dust mites, pet dander, mold spores, and cockroach droppings can trigger or exacerbate asthma symptoms, particularly in individuals with allergic asthma.

- **Irritants:** Respiratory irritants like tobacco smoke, air pollution (including indoor pollution), strong odors, and fumes from cleaning products or chemicals can irritate the airways and contribute to asthma.

- **Respiratory Infections:** Severe respiratory infections, especially during early childhood, have been linked to an increased risk of developing asthma. Viruses like rhinovirus and respiratory syncytial virus (RSV) are common culprits.

- **Occupational Exposures:** Certain occupations that involve exposure to irritants or allergens, such as dust, chemicals, or fumes, can increase the risk of occupational asthma.

3. Immunological Factors:

- **Immune System Dysregulation:** Asthma is, in part, an immune-mediated condition. Individuals with asthma may have immune systems that react abnormally to allergens or irritants, leading to airway inflammation and narrowing.

- **T-helper Cell Imbalance:** An imbalance between T-helper cell subsets, particularly Th1 and Th2 cells, can influence the immune response and may contribute to the development of asthma. Th2-driven responses are often associated with allergic asthma.

4. Early Life Exposures:

- **Early-Life Exposures to Allergens:** Exposure to allergens in infancy and early childhood, when the immune system is still developing, may play a role in sensitizing individuals to these allergens and increasing their risk of developing asthma.

- **Breastfeeding:** Some studies suggest that breastfeeding can reduce the risk of developing asthma in children, possibly due to the protective factors found in breast milk.

5. Obesity:

- Obesity has been associated with an increased risk of asthma, particularly in adults. The exact mechanisms linking obesity and asthma are complex and may involve changes in inflammation and lung function.

It's important to note that asthma is a heterogeneous condition, meaning it can present differently in different individuals. The interplay of genetic predisposition and environmental exposures varies from person to person, which contributes to the diversity in asthma phenotypes.

While the specific causes of asthma are still being explored, understanding these contributing factors can help in developing strategies for prevention, management, and personalized treatment approaches for individuals with asthma.

The Impact on the Lungs

Asthma can have a significant impact on the lungs, as it is a chronic respiratory condition characterized by inflammation and narrowing of the airways. The long-term effects of asthma on the lungs can vary depending on the severity of the condition, how well it is managed, and individual factors. Here's an overview of the impact of asthma on the lungs:

1. Airway Inflammation:

- In asthma, the airways (bronchi and bronchioles) become chronically inflamed. This inflammation is a key feature of the condition and can lead to several consequences.

- Chronic inflammation causes structural changes in the airway walls, including increased thickness and remodeling, which can reduce lung function over time.

2. Bronchoconstriction:

- During asthma attacks or when exposed to triggers, the smooth muscles surrounding the airways can contract excessively. This constriction, known as bronchoconstriction, leads to a narrowing of the airways.

- Bronchoconstriction makes it more difficult for air to flow in and out of the lungs, resulting in the characteristic asthma symptoms of wheezing, coughing, shortness of breath, and

- chest tightness.

3. Reduced Lung Function:

- The combination of airway inflammation and bronchoconstriction can lead to a decline in lung function over time if not properly managed.

- In individuals with uncontrolled or severe asthma, reduced lung function may become a chronic issue, resulting in persistent symptoms and limitations in daily activities.

4. Airway Remodeling:

- Prolonged inflammation and frequent asthma exacerbations can lead to structural changes in the airways, known as airway remodeling. This includes thickening of the airway walls, increased mucus production, and alterations in the connective tissues.

- Airway remodeling can make asthma more resistant to treatment and can contribute to persistent symptoms and airflow obstruction.

5. Risk of Exacerbations:

- People with asthma are at risk of experiencing acute exacerbations or asthma attacks. During an attack, the airways become severely narrowed, making it difficult to breathe. These episodes can be life-threatening if not promptly treated.

- Recurrent asthma attacks can lead to lung damage over time and may contribute to a more severe and chronic form of the condition.

6. Lung Development in Children:

- In children with poorly controlled asthma, the condition can affect lung growth and development. Chronic inflammation and reduced lung function during childhood may lead to long-term consequences for lung health.

7. Risk of Other Lung Conditions:

- Asthma may increase the risk of developing other lung conditions, such as chronic obstructive pulmonary disease (COPD) in adulthood, particularly in individuals who smoke or have significant exposure to respiratory irritants.

It's important to note that with proper asthma management, including appropriate medications and avoidance of triggers, the impact of asthma on the lungs can be minimized. Many individuals with asthma can lead healthy and active lives, maintain good lung function, and prevent exacerbations by following their asthma action plan and working closely with healthcare providers to optimize their treatment. Early diagnosis and effective management are key factors in mitigating the long-term effects of asthma on the lungs.

Chapter 2

The Lung-Healing Diet: Nourishing Your Respiratory System

In our ongoing exploration of the alchemy of asthma, we turn our attention to a critical aspect of managing this condition: the role of diet and nutrition in supporting lung health and mitigating asthma symptoms.

Nutrition plays a crucial role in managing and taking care of asthma. While asthma is primarily a respiratory condition, the foods we eat can have a significant impact on inflammation, immune function, and overall lung health. A well-balanced and nutritious diet can help individuals with asthma reduce symptoms, improve lung function, and

enhance their overall well-being. Here's how the power of nutrition can be harnessed to manage asthma effectively:

Anti-Inflammatory Diet:

- Chronic inflammation of the airways is a central feature of asthma. Consuming an anti-inflammatory diet can help reduce inflammation in the body, including the airways. Such a diet includes:

  - Fruits and vegetables: These are rich in antioxidants, vitamins, and minerals that can help combat inflammation.

  - Omega-3 fatty acids: Found in fatty fish (salmon, mackerel, sardines), flaxseeds, and walnuts, omega-3s have anti-inflammatory properties.

- Foods rich in vitamin D: Vitamin D may have a protective effect against asthma. Sources include fortified dairy products and fatty fish.

2. Magnesium-Rich Foods:

- Magnesium is a mineral that plays a role in relaxing the smooth muscles of the airways. Consuming magnesium-rich foods like nuts, seeds, leafy greens, and whole grains may help reduce bronchoconstriction and asthma symptoms.

3. Antioxidant-Rich Foods:

- Antioxidants, such as vitamins C and E, selenium, and beta-carotene, help combat oxidative stress and reduce airway inflammation. Foods high in antioxidants include berries, citrus fruits, nuts, seeds, and green tea.

4. Maintaining a Healthy Weight:

- Obesity is associated with an increased risk of asthma and may worsen symptoms. Maintaining a healthy weight through a balanced diet and regular physical activity can help improve asthma control.

5. Hydration:

- Staying well-hydrated is important for individuals with asthma. Proper

- hydration helps keep the airway linings moist and can reduce the risk of bronchoconstriction. Water and herbal teas are good choices.

Limiting Trigger Foods:

Certain foods can act as asthma triggers or exacerbate asthma symptoms in some individuals. While not everyone with asthma is affected by food triggers, it's essential to be aware of potential dietary factors that may worsen asthma and to identify any specific triggers for your individual condition. Here are some common asthma trigger foods:

1. **Sulfites:** Sulfites are preservatives added to various foods and drinks to prevent spoilage. Some individuals with asthma may be sensitive to sulfites, which can lead to asthma symptoms. Foods and beverages that may contain sulfites include:

- Wine

- Dried fruits

- Processed potatoes (e.g., French fries)

- Shrimp and other shellfish

- Condiments like vinegar, mustard, and some salad dressings

2. Histamine-Rich Foods: Histamine is a natural compound that can trigger allergy-like symptoms, including respiratory issues, in some people. Foods rich in histamine include:

- Aged cheeses (e.g., cheddar, parmesan)
- Fermented foods (e.g., sauerkraut, yogurt)
- Processed meats (e.g., salami, bacon)
- Some alcoholic beverages (e.g., beer, champagne)

3. Food Allergens: For individuals with both asthma and food allergies, consuming allergenic foods can lead to asthma symptoms as part of an allergic reaction. Common food allergens include:

- Peanuts
- Tree nuts (e.g., almonds, walnuts)
- Shellfish
- Eggs
- Milk
- Wheat
- Soy

4. Food Additives: Some food additives, such as monosodium glutamate (MSG) and artificial food coloring, have been reported as potential asthma triggers in some individuals. These additives are found in various processed foods, so it's important to read food labels carefully if you suspect sensitivity.

5. High-Fat Foods: High-fat and fried foods can contribute to obesity and increase the risk of obesity-related asthma. While not a direct trigger, obesity can worsen asthma symptoms, so it's advisable to maintain a balanced diet.

6. Salicylate-Rich Foods: Salicylates are natural compounds found in some fruits and vegetables, and some people may be sensitive to them. Foods high in salicylates include:

- Tomatoes
- Strawberries
- Apples
- Spinach
- Peppers
- Grapes

7. Cold Drinks and Ice Cream: Extremely cold beverages or ice cream can cause bronchospasms (airway constriction) in some individuals with asthma. This reaction is known as "cold-induced asthma" or "cold air asthma."

8. Food Intolerances: Certain individuals may have food intolerances that lead to digestive symptoms, and in some cases,

these symptoms can indirectly exacerbate asthma symptoms. Common food intolerances include lactose intolerance and gluten sensitivity.

It's important to note that asthma triggers can vary widely from person to person. If you suspect that certain foods may be triggering your asthma symptoms, consider keeping a detailed food diary to track your diet and symptoms. Discuss your concerns with your healthcare provider or an allergist who can help you identify and manage food-related triggers through testing, dietary adjustments, and personalized asthma management plans. In many cases, dietary modifications can help individuals with asthma reduce the risk of symptom exacerbation and improve overall asthma control.

Balanced Macronutrients:

Balanced macronutrients play a crucial role in asthma management, as they can influence inflammation, immune function, and overall respiratory health. A well-rounded diet that includes the right balance of macronutrients—carbohydrates, proteins, and fats—can help individuals with asthma maintain better control of their symptoms and improve lung function. Here's how to ensure a balanced macronutrient intake for asthma management:

1. Carbohydrates:

- **Complex Carbohydrates:** Focus on consuming complex carbohydrates, such as whole grains (e.g., brown rice, quinoa, whole wheat pasta), legumes (e.g., lentils, beans), and fruits and vegetables. These foods provide a steady source of energy and fiber, which can help control blood sugar levels and reduce inflammation.

- **Fiber:** High-fiber foods, like fruits, vegetables, and whole grains, can help maintain a healthy weight and reduce the risk of obesity, which is linked to worsened asthma symptoms.

2. Proteins:

- **Lean Protein Sources:** Opt for lean protein sources like poultry, fish, tofu, legumes, and low-fat dairy products. These provide essential amino acids for muscle health and overall immune function.

- **Omega-3 Fatty Acids:** Fatty fish like salmon, mackerel, and trout are excellent sources of omega-3 fatty acids, which have anti-inflammatory properties. Including these in your diet can help reduce airway inflammation associated with asthma.

3. Fats:

- **Healthy Fats:** Incorporate healthy fats,

- such as those found in avocados, nuts,

  seeds, and olive oil. These fats can help

  reduce inflammation and support

  overall cardiovascular health.

- **Omega-3 Fatty Acids:** As mentioned

  earlier, omega-3 fatty acids from

  sources like fatty fish and flaxseeds can

  have anti-inflammatory effects and

  may benefit individuals with asthma.

4. Hydration:

- **Adequate Fluid Intake:** Staying well-hydrated is essential for individuals with asthma. Proper hydration helps keep mucus thin and makes it easier to clear from the airways. Water is the best choice for hydration, but herbal teas and diluted fruit juices can also be consumed in moderation.

5. Balanced Meals:

- **Balanced Plate:** Aim for balanced meals that include a variety of foods from all food groups. A typical plate should consist of lean protein, complex carbohydrates, and healthy fats, along with plenty of fruits and vegetables.

6. Antioxidants and Vitamins:

- **Fruits and Vegetables:** Colorful fruits and vegetables are rich in antioxidants like vitamin C, vitamin E, and beta-carotene. These antioxidants can help reduce inflammation and protect against oxidative stress, which can trigger asthma symptoms.

7. Avoiding Trigger Foods:

- **Individual Triggers:** Be aware of any specific food triggers that worsen your asthma symptoms. While certain foods are generally beneficial, individual sensitivities can vary.

8. Portion Control:

- **Moderation:** Practice portion control to avoid overeating, which can lead to weight gain and potentially worsen asthma symptoms in some cases.

9. Dietary Restrictions:

- **Consult a Dietitian:** If you have dietary restrictions due to allergies, intolerances, or specific health conditions, consult a registered dietitian for personalized guidance on achieving a balanced macronutrient intake.

Maintaining a balanced diet can complement other aspects of asthma management, such as medication adherence, trigger avoidance, and lifestyle modifications. It's important to work with your healthcare provider and, if necessary, a registered dietitian to develop a comprehensive asthma management plan that includes dietary recommendations tailored to your specific needs and goals.

8. Avoiding Food Allergens:

- In some cases, individuals with asthma may have allergies to certain foods that can exacerbate their symptoms. Common allergenic foods include milk, eggs, peanuts, tree nuts, soy, wheat, fish, and shellfish. Identifying and avoiding these allergens can help improve asthma control.

9. Individualized Nutrition Plan:

- Nutrition needs can vary from person to person, so it's essential to work with a healthcare provider or registered dietitian to create an individualized nutrition plan that takes into account dietary preferences, allergies, and other health conditions.

While nutrition can play a vital role in asthma management, it should be seen as a complementary approach alongside medications and other asthma management strategies. Individuals with asthma should always follow their healthcare provider's guidance, adhere to their prescribed medications, and communicate any dietary changes or concerns with their healthcare team. Properly integrating a nutritious diet into an asthma management plan can contribute to better asthma control and overall well-being.

Chapter 3

Breathing Techniques: Mastering the Art of Relaxation

In the alchemical journey of asthma management, the art of breathing takes center stage in Chapter 3. Here, we delve into the transformative power of various breathing exercises and techniques, offering a pathway to master relaxation and gain control over asthma symptoms.

Breathing is a fundamental and often automatic process, but for individuals with asthma, it can become a source of anxiety and discomfort. Understanding the mechanics of breathing and learning to harness its potential can be a game-changer in managing this condition.

Deep Breathing Exercises

Deep breathing exercises are a valuable technique for individuals with asthma to help improve lung function, reduce stress, and manage their condition more effectively. These exercises can help individuals with asthma learn to use their lung capacity more efficiently, reduce the sensation of breathlessness, and promote relaxation. Here's how deep breathing exercises can benefit those with asthma:

1. Improved Lung Function:

- Deep breathing exercises can enhance lung function by increasing the amount of air that reaches the lower parts of the lungs. This can help individuals with asthma utilize their full lung capacity, which is often compromised due to airway constriction and inflammation.

2. Reduction in Hyperventilation and Breathlessness:

- People with asthma may sometimes experience hyperventilation or rapid, shallow breathing, especially during an asthma attack or when feeling anxious about their symptoms. Deep breathing exercises can help slow down the breathing rate and reduce feelings of breathlessness.

3. Relaxation and Stress Reduction:

- Asthma symptoms can be triggered or exacerbated by stress and anxiety. Deep breathing exercises promote relaxation and can help reduce stress, which may, in turn, help prevent asthma symptoms from worsening.

4. Enhanced Airway Clearance:

- Deep breathing exercises can facilitate the clearance of mucus from the airways. By taking slow, deep breaths, individuals can promote the movement of mucus toward the larger airways, making it easier to clear through coughing.

Here's a simple deep breathing exercise that individuals with asthma can practice:

Diaphragmatic Breathing (Belly Breathing):

1. Find a comfortable, quiet place to sit or lie down.

2. Place one hand on your chest and the other on your abdomen, just below the ribcage.

3. Inhale slowly through your nose, letting your abdomen rise as you fill your lungs with air. Your chest should remain relatively still.

4. Exhale slowly and completely through your mouth, allowing your abdomen to fall.

5. Continue this deep breathing pattern for several minutes, aiming for a slow and steady rhythm.

It's essential to practice deep breathing exercises regularly to incorporate them into your daily routine and experience their full benefits. Some individuals find it helpful to combine deep breathing exercises with techniques like meditation or progressive muscle relaxation for a more comprehensive approach to managing asthma-related stress and anxiety.

While deep breathing exercises can be a valuable tool in asthma management, they should not replace prescribed asthma medications or other treatment recommendations from your healthcare provider. Always consult with your healthcare team to ensure that deep breathing exercises are a safe and suitable addition to your asthma management plan.

The Buteyko Method

The Buteyko Method is a set of breathing exercises and principles designed to respiratory health, reduce symptoms of conditions like asthma, and promote overall well-being. Developed by Russian physiologist Konstantin Buteyko, this method focuses on retraining breathing patterns to optimize oxygenation and reduce the risk of overbreathing, which can lead to various health issues. Here are the steps to practice the Buteyko Method:

1. Find a Comfortable Seated Position:

- Sit in a comfortable chair with your back straight, or you can sit on the floor with your legs crossed. Keep your spine aligned.

2. Relax Your Muscles:

- Close your eyes and relax your facial muscles, shoulders, and neck.

3. Close Your Mouth:

- Keep your mouth closed throughout the practice. This is a fundamental aspect of the Buteyko Method.

4. Breathe Normally for a Few Moments:

- Take a few normal, relaxed breaths through your nose to establish your baseline.

5. Take a Small Breath In:

- Inhale gently and slowly through your nose, taking in a small, comfortable amount of air. Avoid deep or forceful inhalations.

6. Exhale Slowly:

- Exhale slowly and completely through your nose. Focus on maintaining a relaxed exhalation.

7. Pinch Your Nose:

- After your exhalation, pinch your nose closed with your fingers to prevent any air from entering.

8. Hold Your Breath:

- Hold your breath while keeping your mouth closed and holding your nose. The goal is to pause your breath comfortably, not to strain.

9. Pay Attention to Sensations:

- Pay attention to the sensations of air hunger or a slight need to breathe. This is a sign that carbon dioxide levels in your body are increasing, which is a desired effect of the Buteyko Method.

10. Release Your Nose and Exhale: - When you feel a natural urge to breathe or a need to exhale, release your nose and exhale slowly and gently through your nose. Avoid forceful exhalations.

11. Resume Normal Breathing: - Return to normal, relaxed nasal breathing for a minute or two. Notice the difference in your breathing pattern and any sensations of calmness or improved oxygenation.

12. Repeat the Cycle: - Practice this cycle of controlled, shallow breathing followed by breath-holding for a few minutes. Gradually extend the duration as you become more comfortable with the method.

13. Practice Regularly: - Consistency is key to retraining your breathing habits. Aim to practice the Buteyko Method daily, gradually increasing the duration of each session.

14. Monitor Progress: - Over time, you may notice improvements in your breathing pattern, reduced symptoms, and increased tolerance to carbon dioxide. Keep track of your progress to assess the method's effectiveness for you.

15. Seek Guidance if Needed: - If you have a medical condition, especially asthma or other respiratory issues, it's advisable to seek guidance from a qualified Buteyko practitioner or healthcare provider. They can tailor the method to your specific needs and monitor your progress.

The Buteyko Method emphasizes slow, shallow breathing through the nose, which helps maintain healthy carbon dioxide levels in the body. This can have a calming effect on the nervous system and improve overall respiratory health. As with any breathing technique, it's essential to practice mindfully, and if you have any concerns or medical conditions, consult a healthcare professional before beginning the Buteyko Method.

Yoga and Mindful Breathing

Yoga and mindful breathing can be particularly beneficial for individuals with asthma, as they help improve lung function, reduce stress, and enhance overall respiratory health. Here are steps for practicing yoga and mindful breathing specifically for asthma management:

1. Consult Your Healthcare Provider:

- Before starting any new exercise or breathing routine, especially if you have asthma, consult your healthcare provider. They can assess your condition and provide personalized recommendations.

2. Choose a Suitable Yoga Style:

- Opt for a gentle and beginner-friendly yoga style, such as Hatha or Yin yoga, which emphasizes slow, controlled movements and deep breathing. Avoid strenuous or hot yoga classes, which may trigger asthma symptoms.

3. Create a Calm Environment:

- Find a quiet and well-ventilated space for your practice. A calm environment can help reduce stress and promote relaxation.

4. Warm-Up Mindfully:

- Begin your practice with gentle warm-up exercises to prepare your body for yoga poses. Focus on slow, controlled movements and breath awareness.

5. Practice Yoga Poses (Asanas):

- Incorporate a series of yoga poses that emphasize chest and lung opening. Poses like Cobra, Cat-Cow, Bridge, and Child's Pose can be particularly beneficial for asthma. Focus on proper alignment and coordinated breathing.

6. Emphasize Diaphragmatic Breathing:

- Pay special attention to diaphragmatic breathing during your yoga practice. Inhale deeply through your nose, allowing your abdomen to rise, and exhale slowly through your nose, allowing your abdomen to fall.

7. Include Pranayama (Breathing Exercises):

- Integrate specific Pranayama techniques, like Diaphragmatic Breathing, Alternate Nostril Breathing (Nadi Shodhana), and Ocean Breath (Ujjayi), into your yoga routine. These techniques can improve lung capacity and reduce stress.

8. Use Props as Needed:

- If you have limited flexibility or mobility, use yoga props such as blocks, straps, or bolsters to support your practice.

9. Focus on Relaxation:

- Dedicate a portion of your practice to relaxation and stress reduction. Consider incorporating Savasana (Corpse Pose) or a guided meditation.

10. Stay Mindful: - Maintain mindfulness throughout your practice. Be present in each moment, paying attention to your breath and any sensations in your body.

11. Monitor Your Breath: - Keep an eye on your breath and any changes in your breathing pattern. If you notice wheezing or shortness of breath, stop the practice and use your rescue inhaler as needed.

12. Gradually Increase Duration: - Start with shorter practice sessions and gradually increase the duration as your comfort and lung capacity improve.

13. End with Gratitude: - Conclude your practice by expressing gratitude for the opportunity to care for your respiratory health.

14. Carry Mindfulness into Daily Life: - Practice mindful breathing techniques throughout your day, especially during moments of stress or anxiety. Mindful breath awareness can help you manage asthma triggers and symptoms in real-time.

15. Track Your Progress: - Keep a journal to track your asthma symptoms, peak flow measurements, and the impact of your yoga and mindful breathing practice. This can help you assess its effectiveness.

16. Communicate with Your Healthcare Provider: - Regularly update your healthcare provider on your yoga and mindful breathing practice and any changes in your asthma management plan.

17. Be Consistent: - Consistency is key to reaping the full benefits of yoga and mindful breathing for asthma management. Aim to practice regularly, even if it's for a short duration each day.

Remember that yoga and mindful breathing should complement your asthma management plan, which may include medications and other treatments prescribed by your healthcare provider. These practices can empower you to take an active role in managing your asthma and improving your overall quality of life.

Breath Control during Exercise

Breath control during exercise is a critical aspect of asthma management, particularly for individuals with exercise-induced bronchoconstriction (EIB), a condition in which physical activity triggers asthma symptoms. With proper techniques and strategies, individuals with asthma can stay active, improve their fitness, and reduce the risk of exercise-induced asthma symptoms. Here are some key tips for effective breath control during exercise for asthma management:

1. Warm-Up Adequately:

- Before starting strenuous exercise, it's essential to warm up properly. A 10-15 minute warm-up that includes low-intensity aerobic activity can gradually prepare the body for more intense exercise and reduce the likelihood of exercise-induced asthma symptoms.

2. Use Medications as Prescribed:

- For individuals with exercise-induced bronchoconstriction, healthcare providers may prescribe medications like short-acting beta-agonists (e.g., albuterol) to be used before exercise. These medications help relax the airway muscles and can prevent asthma symptoms during physical activity. It's crucial to follow the prescribed dosage and administration instructions.

3. Maintain Proper Technique:

- During exercise, focus on maintaining proper breathing technique. Try to breathe through the nose, as nasal breathing filters, warms, and humidifies the air, reducing the chances of triggering asthma symptoms. When needed, take slow, deep breaths to ensure sufficient oxygen intake.

4. Pacing and Intensity:

- Choose the right level of exercise intensity and pace that suits your fitness level and asthma control. Gradually increase the intensity and duration of exercise over time to build stamina and reduce the risk of sudden asthma symptoms.

5. Stay Hydrated:

- Dehydration can worsen asthma symptoms. Drink plenty of water before, during, and after exercise to stay well-hydrated.

6. Know Your Triggers:

- Be aware of environmental triggers that may worsen asthma symptoms during exercise, such as cold air, pollen, pollution, or allergens. Try to exercise in environments that minimize these triggers or take preventive measures like wearing a mask or using a scarf to warm the air you breathe.

7. Cool Down:

- After exercise, engage in a gradual cool-down period to help your body transition back to its resting state. This can also reduce the risk of post-exercise asthma symptoms.

8. Monitor Symptoms:

- Pay close attention to how your body responds during exercise. If you start to experience asthma symptoms like wheezing, coughing, or shortness of breath, stop exercising and follow your asthma action plan, which may include using a rescue inhaler.

9. Consult a Healthcare Provider:

- It's important to work closely with your healthcare provider to develop an asthma action plan tailored to your needs. Your healthcare provider can help you determine the appropriate medications and dosages for exercise-induced bronchoconstriction and provide guidance on asthma management during physical activity.

10. Choose Asthma-Friendly Activities: - Opt for exercises and activities that are less likely to trigger asthma symptoms. Swimming, cycling, and yoga, for example, are often well-tolerated by individuals with asthma.

Remember that asthma management during exercise is highly individualized. What works for one person may not work for another, so it's essential to consult with your healthcare provider to develop a personalized plan that suits your specific asthma condition and fitness goals. With proper breath control techniques and asthma management strategies, individuals with asthma can lead active and fulfilling lives while minimizing the impact of exercise-induced asthma symptoms.

Personalizing Your Breathing Practice

Personalizing your breathing practice involves tailoring breathing techniques to your individual needs, preferences, and specific goals. Breathing exercises can offer various physical and mental benefits, such as reducing stress, improving lung function, and enhancing relaxation. Here are steps to help you personalize your breathing practice:

1. Understand Your Goals:

- Start by clarifying your objectives. Do you want to reduce stress, improve your focus, manage anxiety, enhance athletic performance, or address specific health concerns like asthma or sleep problems? Knowing your goals will guide your choice of breathing techniques.

2. Consult a Healthcare Professional:

- If you have specific health concerns or medical conditions like asthma, chronic obstructive pulmonary disease (COPD), or anxiety disorders, consult a healthcare professional, such as a doctor or respiratory therapist, for guidance. They can provide personalized recommendations and ensure that your chosen techniques are safe and suitable for your situation.

3. Experiment with Different Techniques:

- There is no one-size-fits-all approach to breathing practices. Explore various techniques, such as diaphragmatic breathing, box breathing, alternate nostril breathing, and mindfulness meditation. Experiment with different techniques to determine which ones resonate with you and align with your goals.

4. Pay Attention to Your Body:

- Be mindful of how your body responds to different breathing practices. Notice the physical sensations, emotions, and changes in your mental state during and after each session. Your body's feedback will help you identify which techniques are most effective for you.

5. Customize Duration and Frequency:

- Adjust the duration and frequency of your breathing practice to fit your schedule and preferences. Some people benefit from short, frequent
- sessions throughout the day, while others prefer longer sessions less frequently. Find a balance that works for you.

6. Incorporate Breathing into Daily Routines:

- Integrate breathing exercises into your daily routines. You can practice mindfulness breathing while commuting, do diaphragmatic breathing before bedtime, or use breath control techniques during workouts.

7. Modify Techniques as Needed:

- Modify breathing techniques to meet your changing needs. For example, if you are using breath control

techniques for anxiety, you may need
different practices during moments of
high stress compared to daily
maintenance.

8. Listen to Guided Sessions:

- Consider using guided breathing
  exercises led by experts. These
  recordings or apps can provide
  structure and guidance as you
  personalize your practice.

9. Keep a Breathing Journal:

- Maintain a journal to track your experiences with different techniques. Note which techniques you enjoyed, which had the most noticeable benefits, and when you practiced. This record can help you refine your personalized practice over time.

10. Seek Feedback: - If you're working with a healthcare professional or therapist, discuss your experiences and progress with them regularly. Their feedback can help you fine-tune your practice.

11. Be Patient and Adaptive: - Understand that personalizing your breathing practice is an ongoing process. It may take time to find the techniques that work best for you, and your needs may change over time. Be flexible and adaptive in your approach.

Remember that the goal of personalizing your breathing practice is to make it a valuable and sustainable part of your daily life. By tailoring your techniques to your unique needs and goals, you can maximize the physical and mental benefits of conscious breathing.

In the alchemy of asthma management, the mastery of breathing techniques is akin to transmuting anxiety and discomfort into a calm and controlled state of being. By embracing these techniques, individuals can take an active role in managing their asthma, fostering relaxation, and achieving a sense of balance on their journey toward better lung health.

Relaxation Techniques during Asthma Attack

Relaxation techniques can be helpful during asthma attacks to manage symptoms and reduce anxiety, which can exacerbate the condition. Asthma is a chronic respiratory condition characterized by inflammation and constriction of the airways, which can lead to symptoms like coughing, wheezing, shortness of breath, and chest tightness. During an asthma attack, it's crucial to both address the physical symptoms and manage the psychological stress and anxiety that often accompany them. Here are some relaxation techniques that can be beneficial during asthma attacks:

1. **Deep Breathing:** Controlled and deep breathing can help calm the nervous system and reduce the feeling of breathlessness. Try the following technique:

- Sit or lie down in a comfortable position.
- Inhale slowly through your nose for a count of 4.
- Hold your breath for a count of 4.
- Exhale slowly and completely through your mouth for a count of 6.
- Repeat this cycle until your breathing becomes more controlled and relaxed.

2. **Pursed-Lip Breathing:** Pursed-lip breathing helps maintain open airways and reduces the effort required to breathe. It can be particularly helpful during an asthma attack:

- Inhale slowly and deeply through your nose.

- Exhale slowly and gently through pursed lips, as if you were blowing out a candle.

- Repeat this pattern to prolong exhalation and prevent rapid breathing.

3. **Progressive Muscle Relaxation:** Tense muscles can make breathing more difficult. Progressive muscle relaxation involves tensing and then releasing different muscle groups to promote relaxation throughout the body. This can help reduce overall tension and anxiety during an asthma attack.

4. **Visualization:** Close your eyes and imagine a peaceful and calming place, such as a beach or a forest. Visualize yourself breathing easily and without any discomfort. Focusing on positive imagery can help reduce stress and anxiety.

5. **Mindfulness and Meditation:** Practicing mindfulness or meditation techniques can help you stay focused on the present moment and reduce panic during an asthma attack. Mindfulness involves paying attention to your breath and body sensations without judgment.

6. **Yoga and Tai Chi:** These gentle, low-impact exercises can help improve lung function, reduce stress, and promote relaxation. Some specific yoga poses and breathing exercises may be particularly helpful for asthma management.

7. **Listening to Calming Music:** Music has a soothing effect and can help distract from the distressing symptoms of an asthma attack. Choose calming and slow-paced music to help reduce anxiety.

8. **Aromatherapy:** Some people find that certain essential oils, like lavender or eucalyptus, can help promote relaxation and open airways. Use a diffuser or inhale the aroma of the essential oil (diluted properly) during an asthma attack.

It's essential to remember that relaxation techniques should complement, not replace, prescribed asthma medications and medical advice from your healthcare provider. If you're experiencing an asthma attack, use your prescribed rescue inhaler and seek immediate medical attention if symptoms do not improve or worsen. Additionally, discuss the use of relaxation techniques with your healthcare provider to ensure they are safe and appropriate for your specific asthma management plan.

Chapter 4

Medications and Treatment Options

In the alchemical process of managing asthma, Chapter 4 serves as a vital crucible, where we explore the array of medications and treatment options available. These tools, when used wisely, have the power to transform the experience of asthma, offering relief, control, and the promise of a better quality of life.

The Asthma Medication Toolbox

Asthma medications are divided into two main categories: long-term control medications and quick-relief medications. Each serves a distinct role in managing the condition, working together to provide optimal asthma control.

Long-Term Control Medications

1. **Inhaled Corticosteroids (ICS):** These are the cornerstone of asthma treatment. ICS reduce airway inflammation and are typically used daily to prevent asthma symptoms. They are safe when used as directed but may have side effects if not taken as prescribed.

2. **Long-Acting Beta-Agonists (LABAs):** LABAs are often used in combination with ICS to help open the airways and maintain symptom control. They should never be used as a stand-alone medication for asthma.

3. **Leukotriene Modifiers:** These medications block leukotrienes, substances that contribute to inflammation in the airways. They are available in pill form and are suitable for some individuals, particularly those who have difficulty with inhalers.

4. **Biologics:** For severe asthma cases, biologic medications can target specific immune system components involved in asthma. These treatments are administered via injection or infusion and are reserved for those with uncontrolled asthma despite other therapies.

Quick-Relief Medications

1. **Short-Acting Beta-Agonists (SABAs):** SABAs provide rapid relief during asthma attacks by relaxing the airway muscles, making it easier to breathe. They are often used as a rescue medication.

Combination Medications

Some medications combine long-acting bronchodilators and corticosteroids in one inhaler. These are beneficial for individuals who require both types of medication for asthma control.

Other Treatment Options

In addition to medications, several other treatments and strategies can enhance asthma management:

1. **Allergen Immunotherapy:** This treatment involves exposure to allergens in a controlled manner, aiming to reduce sensitivity and allergic asthma triggers over time.

2. **Asthma Action Plan:** An individualized plan created with your healthcare provider that outlines how to manage asthma, including medication use and actions to take during an asthma attack.

3. **Lifestyle Modifications:** Avoiding asthma triggers, maintaining a healthy weight, regular exercise, and proper hydration can complement medication management.

4. **Breathing Exercises:** As discussed in Chapter 4, various breathing techniques can help manage asthma symptoms and improve lung function.

Potential Side Effects

All medications come with potential side effects, and it's crucial to be aware of these when managing asthma:

- Inhaled corticosteroids, when used properly, usually have minimal side effects but may include throat irritation or oral fungal infections.

- Long-acting beta-agonists can increase the risk of severe asthma exacerbations if not used in combination with an inhaled corticosteroid.

- Leukotriene modifiers may cause mood changes, headache, and other side effects.

- Biologics may have rare but serious side effects, so close monitoring is essential.

Collaborative Care

Effective asthma management often requires a collaborative effort between individuals with asthma, their healthcare providers, and possibly specialists. Regular follow-ups, open communication, and adjustments to the treatment plan as needed are essential to achieving optimal asthma control.

Chapter 5

Natural Remedies and Alternative Therapies

In our ongoing quest to explore the alchemy of asthma management, Chapter 5 shines a spotlight on natural remedies and alternative therapies. These holistic approaches offer additional tools for individuals seeking a well-rounded and personalized strategy to manage asthma and promote overall lung health.

The Holistic Perspective

Holistic approaches to asthma management view the individual as a whole, considering physical, emotional, and environmental factors that may influence the condition.

While not intended as a replacement for standard medical treatments, these alternative therapies can complement conventional asthma management strategies.

Acupuncture

Acupuncture, an ancient Chinese practice, involves the insertion of thin needles into specific points on the body to stimulate energy flow. Some people with asthma find relief from symptoms through acupuncture, as it may help reduce inflammation, improve lung function, and promote relaxation. It's essential to seek out a qualified acupuncturist who specializes in respiratory conditions.

Herbal Remedies

Herbal remedies have been used for centuries in various cultures to manage respiratory conditions. Certain herbs, such as ginger, turmeric, and licorice root, have anti-inflammatory properties that may benefit individuals with asthma. However, it's crucial to consult with a healthcare provider before incorporating herbal remedies into your asthma management plan, as they can interact with medications and may not be suitable for everyone.

Homeopathy

Homeopathy is a system of alternative medicine that uses highly diluted substances to stimulate the body's natural healing mechanisms. Some individuals with asthma turn to homeopathic remedies, but scientific evidence supporting their effectiveness is limited. It's crucial to consult with a healthcare provider before using homeopathic treatments.

Dietary Modifications

Diet plays a significant role in asthma management, as discussed in Chapter 2. By making thoughtful dietary choices and potentially incorporating anti-inflammatory foods, individuals can complement their asthma management plan with a natural, nutrition-based approach.

The Importance of Consultation

Before embarking on any natural remedy or alternative therapy, it is vital to consult with a healthcare provider or specialist who can provide guidance and assess the appropriateness of these approaches for your specific asthma needs. Some natural remedies may interact with medications or exacerbate asthma symptoms, so informed decision-making is essential.

In the alchemy of asthma management, natural remedies and alternative therapies serve as additional tools in the toolkit, offering holistic perspectives and personalized approaches to enhancing lung health. By incorporating these practices under the guidance of healthcare professionals, individuals can further transform their experience of asthma, fostering well-being and balance on their journey to better lung health.

Chapter 6

Environmental Triggers: Clearing the Air

Asthma is a complex condition influenced by various factors, and one of the most significant contributors to asthma symptoms is the environment. In this chapter, we will explore the common environmental triggers of asthma and discuss strategies to minimize exposure. By understanding and addressing these triggers, you can take proactive steps to manage your asthma effectively and improve your overall quality of life.

Environmental triggers are substances or conditions in the environment that can exacerbate asthma symptoms or even trigger asthma attacks. These triggers vary from person to person, but some are more common than others. It's essential to identify and manage these triggers to maintain good asthma control.

Common Environmental Asthma Triggers:

1. **Allergens**
2. **Irritants**
3. **Respiratory Infections**
4. **Occupational Exposures**

To delve deeper into the specifics of asthma triggers, please refer to Chapter 1.

Minimizing Exposure to Environmental Triggers

Now that we've identified common environmental asthma triggers, let's discuss strategies to minimize exposure:

1. **Allergen Control:**

   - Use allergen-proof covers on pillows and mattresses to reduce exposure to dust mites.

   - Wash bedding regularly in hot water.

   - Maintain a clean and clutter-free home to minimize dust accumulation.

   - Control indoor humidity levels to prevent mold growth.

- Regularly clean and vacuum carpets, rugs, and upholstered furniture.
- Consider using air purifiers with HEPA filters to remove allergens from the air.

2. **Smoke-Free Environment:**

- If you smoke, quit. Smoking worsens asthma and is a major health risk.
- Avoid exposure to secondhand smoke by creating a smoke-free home and workplace.

3. **Air Quality Management:**

- Stay informed about outdoor air quality levels, especially during high pollution days. Limit outdoor activities on poor air quality days.

- Ensure proper ventilation when cooking to minimize indoor air pollution.

- Use exhaust fans in bathrooms and kitchens to reduce humidity and prevent mold growth.

4. Pet Care:

- If you have asthma triggered by pet dander, consider finding a new home for your pet or keeping them outside. If that's not an option, create pet-free zones in your home.

- Bathe and groom pets regularly to reduce dander.

5. Infection Prevention:

- Practice good hand hygiene, especially during cold and flu seasons.

- Get recommended vaccinations, including the annual flu shot.

- Avoid close contact with individuals who have respiratory infections.

6. Occupational Asthma:

- If you suspect your workplace is causing or exacerbating your asthma, consult with your employer and healthcare provider. Occupational asthma may require workplace modifications or changes.

Remember that asthma management is highly individualized. Identifying and addressing environmental triggers is a crucial step in achieving good asthma control. Work closely with your healthcare provider to develop an asthma action plan that includes strategies for managing environmental triggers. By taking these proactive measures, you can reduce the impact of environmental triggers on your asthma and enjoy a healthier, more comfortable life.

Chapter 7

Empowering Yourself: Living Well with Asthma

As we approach the culmination of our exploration into the alchemy of asthma management, Chapter 7 serves as a beacon of empowerment—a guide to living well with asthma. This chapter offers practical tips, tools, and a mindset shift to help individuals take control of their asthma management and lead fulfilling lives.

The Power of Knowledge

1. **Educate Yourself:** Knowledge is a potent tool in asthma management. Learn about your condition, treatment options, and triggers. Stay informed about the latest research and guidelines.

2. **Asthma Action Plan:** Work with your healthcare provider to create and regularly update an asthma action plan. This plan outlines steps to take in various situations, empowering you to make informed decisions.

Lifestyle and Self-Care

3. **Healthy Lifestyle:** Maintain a balanced diet, engage in regular exercise (as tolerated), prioritize sleep, and manage stress. A healthy lifestyle can improve lung function and overall well-being.

4. **Hydration:** Stay well-hydrated to keep airways moist and reduce mucus buildup.

5. **Medication Adherence:** Take your medications as prescribed. Adherence to your treatment plan is vital for asthma control.

Triggers and Environmental Control

6. **Identify Triggers:** Be vigilant in identifying and minimizing asthma triggers, whether they are allergens, irritants, or stressors.

7. **Clean Air:** Ensure good indoor air quality by using air purifiers, maintaining ventilation, and reducing exposure to tobacco smoke and other pollutants.

8. **Allergen Reduction:** Implement measures to reduce allergens in your home, such as using allergen-proof covers for bedding and regular cleaning.

Regular Monitoring

9. **Peak Flow Monitoring:** If recommended by your healthcare provider, use a peak flow meter to monitor your lung function regularly. This can help identify changes in asthma control.

10. **Regular Check-Ups:** Maintain regular appointments with your healthcare provider to assess your asthma, adjust treatment plans, and address any concerns.

Empowering Mindset

11. **Advocacy:** Be an advocate for yourself by communicating openly with your healthcare team and seeking the best care for your asthma.

12. **Mindfulness and Resilience:** Embrace mindfulness practices, such as meditation and deep breathing exercises, to manage stress and cultivate resilience.

13. **Support Network:** Build a strong support network that includes family, friends, and support groups. Sharing experiences and seeking support can be empowering.

Education and Awareness

14.   **Educate Others:** Help those around you understand asthma, its triggers, and how to respond during an asthma attack. This knowledge can be invaluable in emergency situations.

15.   **Raise Awareness:** Participate in asthma awareness initiatives to promote understanding and support for those living with the condition.

Embracing Life with Asthma

16.   **Pursue Your Passions:** Asthma should not limit your aspirations. Pursue your interests, hobbies, and goals with the understanding that

asthma management can empower rather than hinder.

17. **Travel and Adventure:** Plan travel and outdoor activities with asthma in mind. Ensure you have necessary medications, a copy of your asthma action plan, and knowledge of nearby healthcare facilities.

Never Stop Learning

Asthma management is a lifelong journey, and it is crucial to remain curious, adaptable, and proactive. Seek out new information, technologies, and therapies that can enhance your asthma control and quality of life.

In the alchemy of asthma management, empowerment is the final, transformative phase. By implementing these tips and tools and embracing a proactive mindset, you can take charge of your asthma, minimize its impact on your life, and embark on a fulfilling journey towards better lung health and well-being.

Conclusion

As we conclude our journey through the pages of "Asthma Alchemy: Transforming Your Lung Health," we arrive at a destination far more profound than the sum of its chapters. This book has been a guide, a companion, and a source of empowerment on your quest to conquer asthma, transform your lung health, and reclaim the vitality and well-being that are rightfully yours.

Throughout these chapters, we have explored the intricate nature of asthma, unraveled its mysteries, and laid bare its challenges. We've delved into the science of asthma, dissected its triggers, and examined the art of asthma management.

But beyond the knowledge and strategies, "Asthma Alchemy" is a testament to the human spirit's capacity to adapt, to overcome, and to transform adversity into strength. It underscores the vital importance of taking charge of your asthma management, partnering with healthcare providers, and embracing a proactive mindset.

As you close this book, remember that your asthma alchemy journey is ongoing. It is a journey of empowerment, resilience, and the pursuit of a fulfilling life with better lung health. Continue to educate yourself, advocate for your well-being, and seek support from your community and healthcare team.

You have the power to transform your relationship with asthma, turning it from a burden into an opportunity for growth and better health. May the lessons and insights shared within these pages accompany you on your path to breathing easier, living healthier, and discovering the alchemical art of transforming your lung health.

Your journey is not ending here; it is just beginning, and the possibilities for a brighter, healthier future are limitless. So, embrace your newfound empowerment, and let your asthma alchemy continue to shape a life of vitality, well-being, and fulfillment.

www.ingramcontent.com/pod-product-compliance
Lightning Source LLC
Chambersburg PA
CBHW070937260726
48661CB00003B/1027